The Guide to Underst Nutritional Value of Fruits and Vegetables

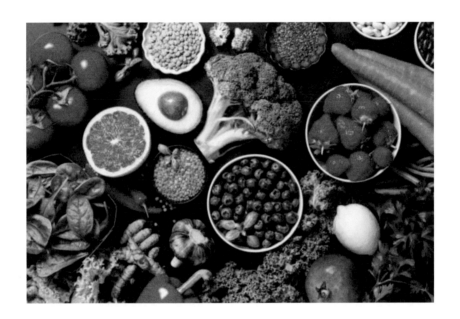

By Nadine Muhammad, MS

Allah (God) in the Person of Master Fard Muhammad, has taught me that fasting and the right kind of food are the cures to our ills. He has told me there is no cure in drugs and medicine. And this, the world is now learning. We can take medicine all of our lives until it kills us, but we are still ailing with the same old diseases (Muhammad, 1972).

"Let thy food be thy medicine and medicine be thy food" (Hippocrates).

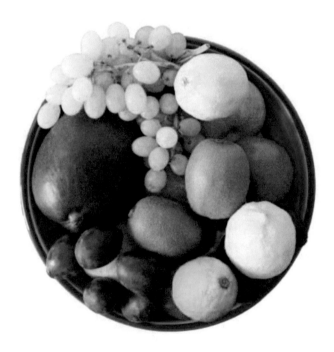

Fruits & Vegetables

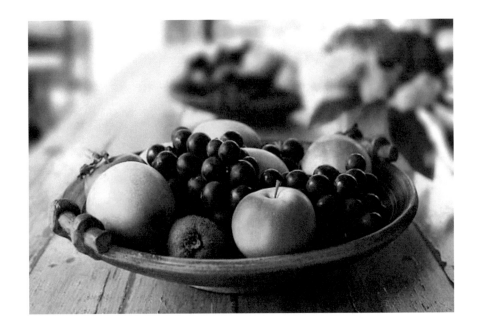

Apples

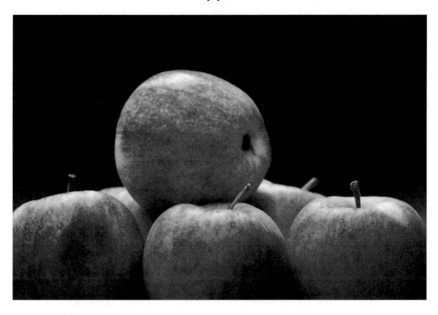

Source Of:

Carbohydrates: Carbohydrate: 14.8 g   Fiber: 2 g Sugar: 12 g

Minerals: Calcium: 5 mg

Magnesium: 4.7 mg Potassium: 95 mg

Vitamins: Vitamin B-6: 0.021 mg

Health Benefits:

Helps in preventing constipation. Apples support digestion, brain health and weight management. "Several studies have specifically linked to apple consumption with a reduced risk for cancer, especially lung cancer. A reduced risk of cardiovascular disease has been associated with apple consumption (Boyer & Liu, 2004).

Avocado

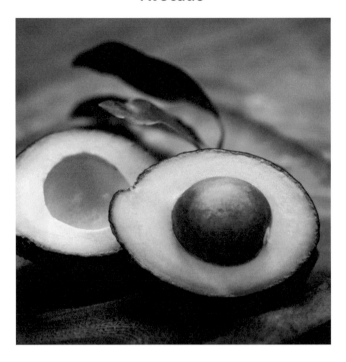

Source of:

Carbohydrates: Carbohydrate: 8 g Fiber: 6 g

Minerals: Calcium: 12 mg; Magnesium: 29 mg Phosphorus: 52 mg Potassium: 485

Vitamins: Vitamin C:10 mg

Health Benefits:

Avocados are good for your skin. Also, they are good for digestion, heart and joint health. Several studies have demonstrated the health benefits of a balanced diet with avocado intake, especially in lowering cholesterol and preventing cardiovascular diseases. (Duarte et al., 2016).

Bananas

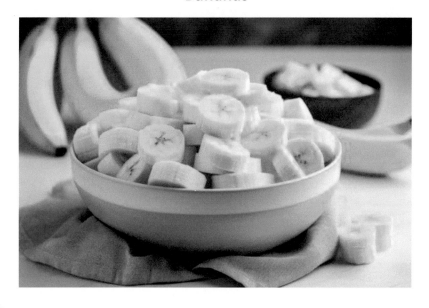

Source of:

Carbohydrates: Carbohydrate: 21 g Fiber: 2 g Sugar: 15.8 g

Minerals: Calcium: 5mg Magnesium: 28 mg Phosphorus 22 mg Potassium: 326 mg

Vitamins: Vitamin C: 12.3 Folate: 14: mcg

Health Benefits:

Bananas aid in the body's retention of calcium, nitrogen, and phosphorus, all of which work to build healthy and regenerated tissues. Potassium benefits the muscles as it helps maintain their proper working and prevents muscle spasms. recent studies are showing that potassium can help to decrease blood pressure in individuals who are potassium deficient. Potassium also reduces the risk of stroke (Singh, et al., 2016).

Blueberries

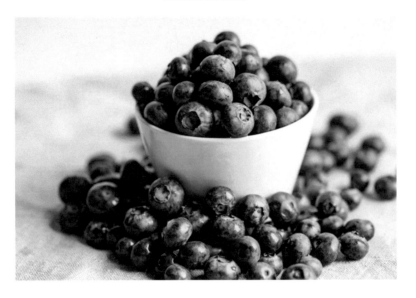

Source Of:

Carbohydrates: Carbohydrate: 14.6 g Sugars: 9.3 g

Minerals: Calcium: 12 mg Potassium 86 mg

Vitamins: Vitamin C: 8.1 mg

Health Benefits:

Blueberry is known as a healthy fruit, mainly because it is rich in anthocyanins. Accumulating research has shown that anthocyanins from the small blue fruits of blueberry plants have important nutritional and health value. In addition to their well-known antioxidant effects, blueberry anthocyanins, which are among the predominant active ingredients, also have relatively good anti-type 2 diabetes, anti-cardiovascular disease, anti-inflammatory and anti-cancer effects (Wu et al, 2023).

Cherry

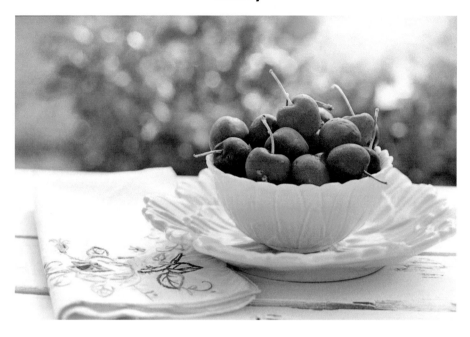

Source Of:

Carbohydrates: Carbohydrate: 16.2 g Sugars: 13.9

Minerals: Calcium: 12 mg Magnesium: 12.1 mg Phosphorus: 23 mg Potassium: 230 mg

Vitamins: Vitamin C: 10.4 mg Vitamin B-6: 0.049 mg

Health Benefits:

Results from studies demonstrated that consumption of fresh cherries prevented attacks of arthritis and restored the plasma uric acid (UA) concentrations to normal levels in all 12 patients. Also, "research results suggest that consumption of sweet or tart cherries can promote health by preventing or decreasing oxidative stress and inflammation (Kelley et al., 2018).

Dates, Medjool

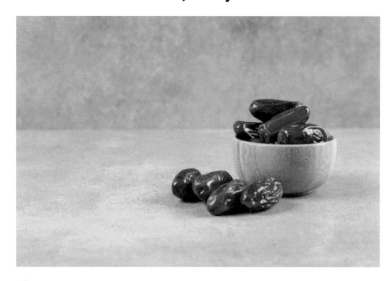

Source Of:

Carbohydrates: Carbohydrate: 75 g Fiber: 6.7 g Sugars: 66.5 g

Minerals: Calcium: 64 mg Magnesium: 54 mg Potassium: 696 mg

Vitamins: Vitamin A: 149 UI Vitamin K: 2.7 ug

Health Benefits:

Dates have a high nutritional value and are rich in carbohydrates, dietary fibers, proteins, minerals, and many vitamins including B complex. Carbohydrates comprise 70% of dates mainly as fructose and glucose in addition, dates are rich in calcium, iron, magnesium, selenium, copper, phosphorus, potassium, zinc, sulfur, cobalt, fluorine, and manganese. Recently, there has been enhanced interest in the abundant health-promoting properties of dates. Dates provide antioxidant, anti-inflammatory, gastrointestinal-protection, and anticancer properties that are vital for human health (Tang et al., Citation2013). In addition, consumption of dates could help to reduce and control diabetes mellitus and other cardio-and cerebrovascular diseases (CCVD) (Tang et al., Citation2013). Lastly, the high potassium and low sodium content in dates are beneficial for people suffering from hypertension (Ayad et.al, 2020).

Fig

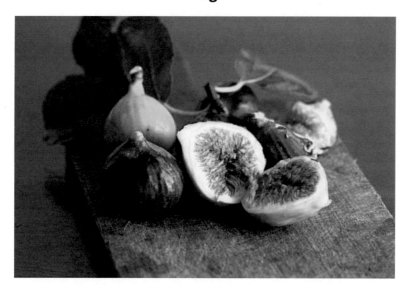

Source of:

Carbohydrates: Carbohydrate: 63.9 g Fiber: 9.8 g Sugars: 47.9 g

Minerals: Calcium: 162 mg Iron: 2.3 mg Magnesium: 67.6 mg Phosphorus: 67 mg Potassium: 680 mg Sodium: 10 mg Zinc: 0.66 mg

Vitamins: Vitamin C: 1.2 mg   Vitamin B-6: 0.106 mg Folate: 9 mcg

Health Benefits:

Fig fruit is an excellent source of water-soluble vitamin C, known as a natural antioxidant, and helps in preventing the nonenzymatic browning of fruits and vegetables. It is utilized as a substitute for synthetic antioxidants. The vitamin plays a vital role in the immune reaction, detoxification, iron absorption, wound healing, orthogenesis, collagen biosynthesis, preventing the blood vessels from clotting, and in various metabolic processes. The research has shown that fig fruit additionally reveals an extremely good composition of bioactive compounds. In vivo and in vitro experiments on human molecular strains together with the animal version the usage of fig fruit/leaves extract has proved its useful impact as anticancer, antidiabetic, antioxidant, antimicrobial, and anti-inflammatory. Figs also help in managing various skin conditions as it has a moisturizing effect which helps in reducing hyperpigmentation, acne, and wrinkles. It can help in making beauty products and figs can also be used for strengthening and improving hair quality (Walia, 2022).

Grapes -Green

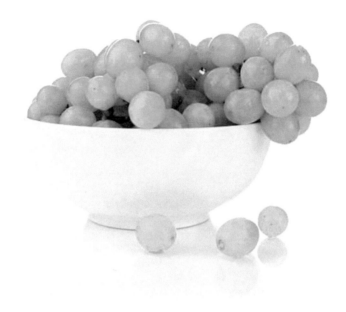

Source of:

Carbohydrates: Carbohydrate: 18.6 g   Sugars: 16.1 g

Minerals: Calcium: 10 mg Iron: 0.2 mg Magnesium: 7.1 mg   Phosphorus: 22 mg   Potassium: 218 mg

Vitamins: Vitamin C: 3 mg

Health Benefits:

Grapes contain a variety of nutrients offering a good supply of calcium, magnesium, potassium, vitamin K, and other important nutrients for bone health. This decreases the risk of fractures and breakage of bones as the likelihood of bone injuries increases without these nutrients. Vitamin C, necessary for boosting immunity, is present in one cup of grapes. Our bodies cannot naturally generate Vitamin C. Therefore, it is crucial to consume foods rich in vitamin C to compensate. Grapes' inherent antibacterial properties, which guard against bacteria and viruses, also help to boost your immune system (Daub, 2022).

Oranges

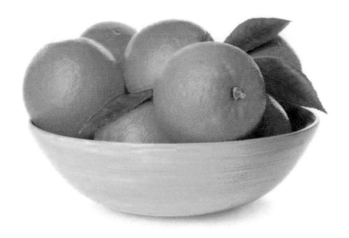

Source of:

Carbohydrates: Carbohydrate: 11.8 g Sugars: 8.57 g

Minerals: Calcium: 43 mg Magnesium: 10.7 mg Phosphorus: 23 mg Potassium: 166 mg

Vitamins: Vitamin C: 59.1 mg   Vitamin B-6: 0.079 mg

Health Benefits:

Numerous therapeutic properties have been attributed to citrus fruits, such as oranges like anticancer, antiviral, anti-tumor, anti-inflammatory activities, and effects on capillary fragility as well as an ability to inhabit platelet aggregation. Benefits of citrus fruits are linked to the high amounts of photochemical and bioactive compounds such as flavonoids, carotenoids, vitamins and minerals available in citrus fruits. These phytonutrients may act as antioxidants, stimulate the immune systems; induce protective enzymes in the liver (Okwu, 2008).

Kiwi

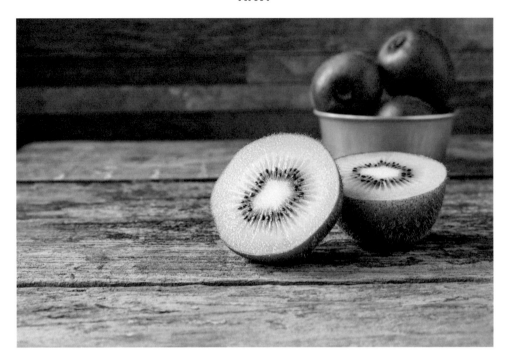

Source of:

Carbohydrates: Carbohydrate: 12 g   Fiber: 3 g Sugars: 8.99 g

 Minerals: Calcium: 35 mg   Magnesium: 15.7 mg   Phosphorus: 34 mg Potassium: 198 mg Sodium: 5 mg

Vitamins: Vitamin C: 74.7 mg

Health Benefits:

It is a good source of vitamin C which is essential nutrient that works in our bodies as an antioxidant to help prevent damage caused by the sun, pollution and smoke, smooth wrinkles, keep the skin young, vibrant and improve overall skin texture. It also a good source of vitamin E which makes the skin soft and moist and protect the skin from degeneration. Folate, magnesium and Vitamin E are all well represented in kiwifruit, offering health benefits that range from bone formation. Vitamin K also has a role in the bone mass building by promoting osteotrophic activity in the bone. Lastly, the fiber and potassium in kiwis support heart health. Fiber can reduce high cholesterol levels, which may reduce the risk of heart disease and heart attack" (Tyagi, et al., 2015).

Melon -Cantaloupe

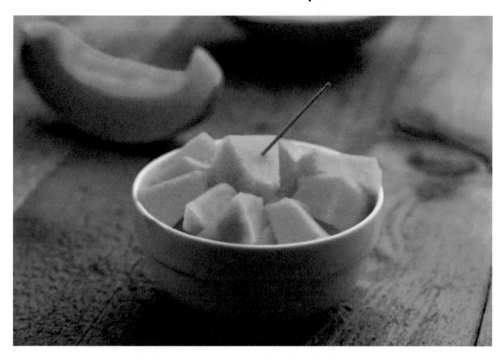

Source of:

Carbohydrates: Carbohydrate:8 g Sugars 7 g

Minerals: Calcium :9 mg Magnesium mg Phosphorus: 17 mg Potassium: 157 mg Sodium 30 mg

Vitamins: Vitamin C: 10 mg

Health Benefits:

A previous study shows that cantaloupe pulp extract possesses high antioxidant and anti-inflammatory properties. Srokka and Cisowski, (2023) Phenolic compounds such as, quercetin and ellagic acid contained in cantaloupe, are good antioxidants that are able to protect body cells from injuries caused by reactive oxygen and nitrogen species (Ismail et al., 2010).

Melon-Honey Dew Melon

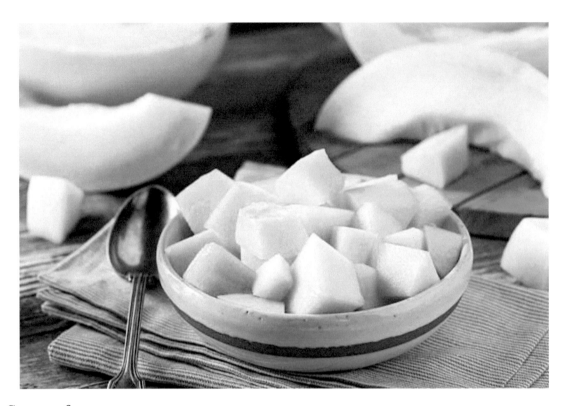

Source of:

Carbohydrates: Carbohydrate: 8 g Sugars 7 g

Minerals: Calcium :9 mg   Magnesium 10 mg Phosphorus: 17 mg   Potassium: 157 mg Sodium: 30 mg

Vitamins: Vitamin C: 10 mg

Health Benefits:

Honeydew is rich in folic acid, thiamine, and riboflavin. Vitamin C and pro-vitamin A are abundantly present in it. Ivanova, states "this is recommended mainly in the case of anemia, atherosclerosis, gout, rheumatism, cardiovascular, kidney, and liver diseases (Khalid et al., 2021).

Melon-Watermelon

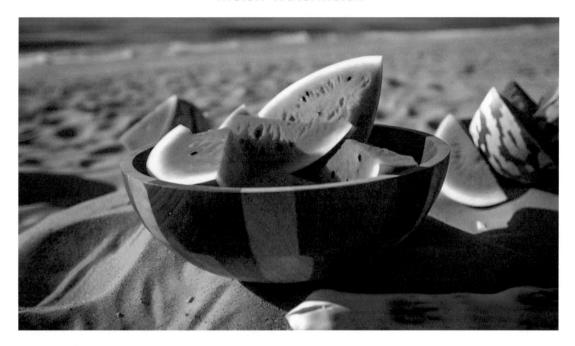

Source Of:

Carbohydrates: Carbohydrate: 7 g Sugars 6g

Minerals: Calcium :7 mg   Magnesium 10 mg Phosphorus: 11 mg   Potassium: 112 mg Sodium: 1mg

Vitamins: Vitamin C: 8 mg

Healthy Benefits:

Watermelon contains phytochemicals such as lycopene, vitamin C, β-carotene, and total polyphenolic content that possess anti-inflammatory, anticancer, and antioxidant properties. Dietary intake of watermelon provides antioxidants properties which is important in maintaining health and well-being. They reduce incidence of chronic diseases such as hypertension, diabetes, cancer, and some coronary heart diseases, through inhibiting formation of free radicals and reactive oxygen species (Maoto, 2019).

Nectarine

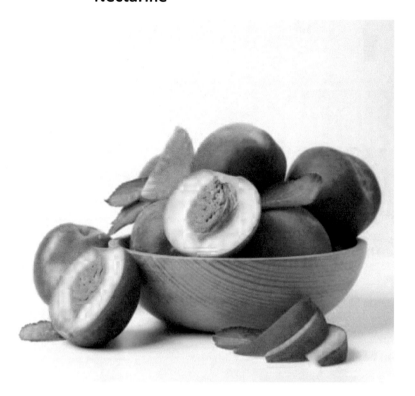

Source Of:

Carbohydrates: Carbohydrate: 79 g Sugars 7 g

 Minerals: Calcium :2 mg   Magnesium 9 mg Phosphorus: 26 mg Potassium: 31 mg
Sodium: 1 mg

Vitamins: Vitamin C: 4 mg

Health Benefits:

Nectarines are juicy, delicious fruits having low calorific value and have high antioxidant
capacity. Its fruits contain fairly good amount of antioxidant vitamins such as C, A, E and
flavonoid polyphenolic antioxidants like lutien, zeaxanthin and β-cryptoxanthin (Colaric
et al. 2005). Further, nectarines are juicy, delicious fruits having low calorific value (44
calories/100 g pulp) and have high antioxidant capacity which prevents oxidative stress
by suppressing the ROS production in human plasma. Hence the consumption of
nectarines which is now considered as functional food is inevitable as it provides
protection from chronic diseases (Jayarajan,2019).

Peach

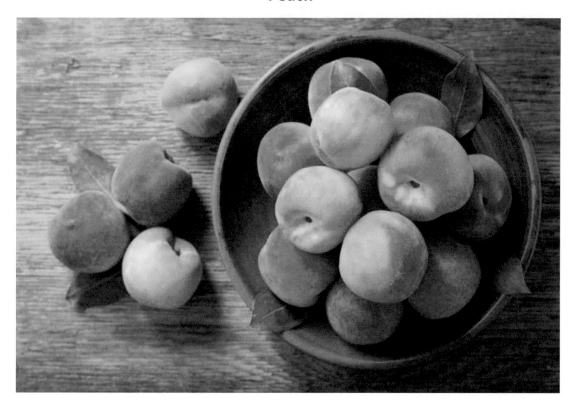

Source of:

Carbohydrates: Carbohydrate: 9 g

Minerals: Calcium: 4 mg   Magnesium 8 mg Phosphorus: 22 mg   Potassium: 122 mg Sodium: 13 mg

Vitamins: Vitamin C: 2 mg

Health Benefits:

The phenolic compounds in peaches have been found to play important roles due to their antioxidant, antimicrobial and anti-inflammatory properties. Evidence has risen about their preventive effects on multiple chronic and age-related diseases such as diabetes, obesity, hypertension, inflammation, cardiovascular, neurodegenerative and oncologic diseases. A variety of studies have focused on testing and determining the phenolic content of peach extracts, which have shown great potential as free-radical scavengers and providing protection against several chronic/age-related diseases (Bento, 2022).

Pears

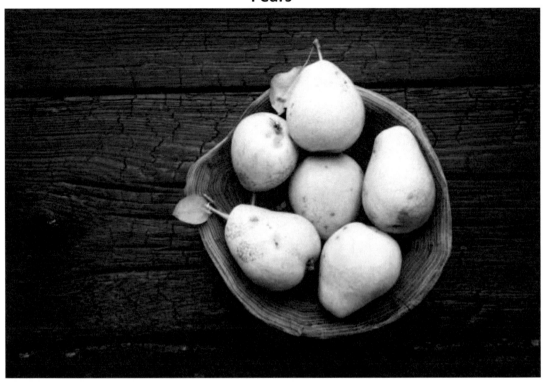

Source Of:

Carbohydrates: Carbohydrate: 15 g Fiber: 6 mg

 Minerals: Calcium :8 mg   Magnesium 5 mg Phosphorus: 10 mg   Potassium: 87 mg
Sodium: 7g

Vitamins: Vitamin C: 4mg

Health Benefits:

Pears are an excellent source of dietary fiber and a good source of vitamin C. Pears, like
most fruit, provide potassium to the diet. Dietary fiber and potassium are nutrients of
concern in the US diet pears are rich in fructose and sorbitol. In combination with dietary
fiber, consumption of pears should improve gut health and prevent constipation. Pears
provide antioxidants and are concentrated in flavanols, particularly anthocyanins. Intake
of pears/apples in prospective cohort studies is linked to less type 2 diabetes and stroke.
The body of evidence for a relationship between pear intake and health outcomes is
sparse and diverse (Reiland & Slavin, 2015).

Pineapple

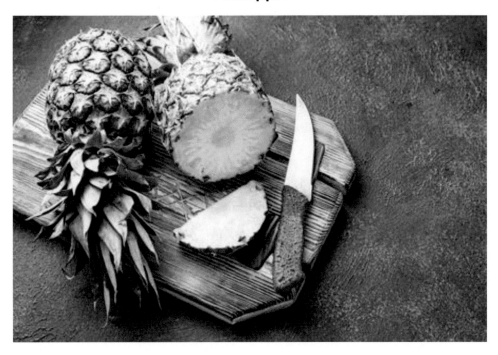

Source Of:

Carbohydrates: Carbohydrate: 14 g Sugar: 11 g

Minerals: Calcium: 12 mg   Magnesium 13 mg Phosphorus: 5 mg   Potassium: 137 mg Sodium: 13 mg

Vitamins: Vitamin C: 58 mg

Health Benefits:

Pineapples are particularly rich in flavonoids and phenolic acids known as antioxidants. Several studies have shown pineapple and its compounds can reduce cancer risk. This is because oxidative stress and inflammation can be minimized. Eating pineapples will reduce the amount of time needed to recover from surgery or exercise. This is primarily due to the bromelain's anti-inflammatory properties. Excessive inflammation is often associated with cancer (Mohsin,2020).

Raspberry

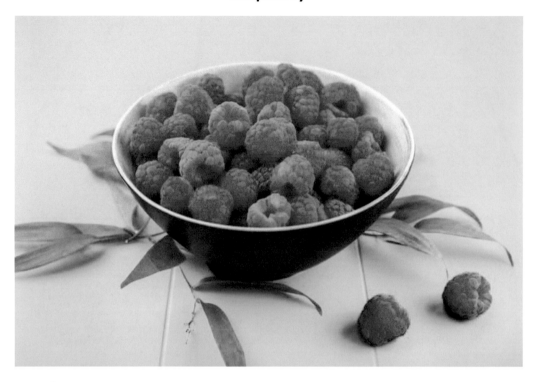

Source of:

Carbohydrates: Carbohydrate: 12 g Fiber: 6 mg Sugar 2 g

 Minerals: Calcium: 16 mg   Magnesium 19 mg Phosphorus: 27 mg   Potassium: 156 mg Sodium 7mg

Vitamins: Vitamin C: 23 mg

Health Benefits:

Raspberries hold a special position among the berries due to their ideal nutritional profile of low calories, fat, and saturated fats, high fiber, presence of several essential micronutrients, and phytochemical composition. They contain a whole range of polyphenolic antioxidant compounds that play a significant role in mitigating the damaging effects of oxidative stress on cells and reducing the risk of chronic diseases (Rao and Snyder, 2010).

Strawberry

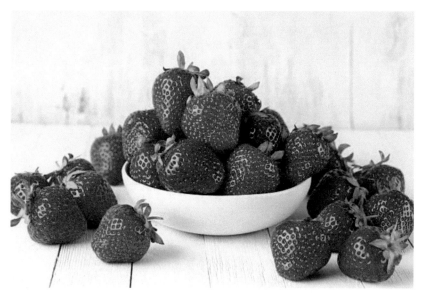

Source Of:

Carbohydrates: Carbohydrate: 7 g   Sugar: 4 g

Minerals: Calcium: 17 mg Magnesium: 12 mg Potassium: 161 mg   Phosphorus: 23 mg

Vitamins: Vitamin C: 59 mg

Health Benefits:

The strawberry represents a healthy food choice. First of all, its dietary fiber and fructose contents may contribute in regulating blood sugar levels by slowing digestion, with its fiber content also contributing to control calorie intake by its satiating effect" (Giampieri et al., 2012). Among strawberry micronutrients, the level of vitamin C is generally considered as a parameter of particular interest for the nutritional evaluation of strawberry varieties, and is often included in the pool of chemical measurements conducted for screening purposes and for the evaluation of the breeding strategies. However, also folate plays a crucial role in emphasizing the nutritional value of a strawberry, when considering that the fruit is among the richest natural food sources of folate" The term folate refers to a wide group of derivatives of the water-soluble B vitamin (tetrahydrofolic acid) much more frequent in food and in the human body than the more stable synthetic form, folic acid, used as supplement and in food fortification (Tulipan et. al. 2009).

Grapefruit

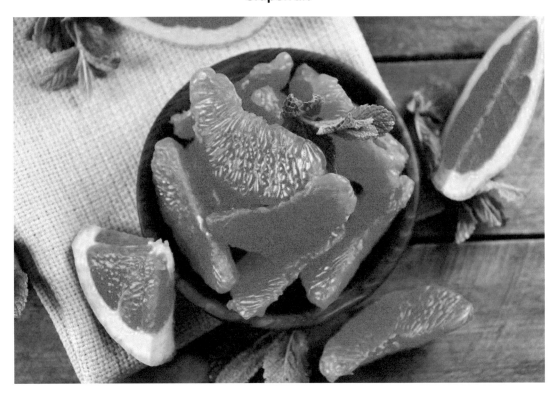

Source Of:

Carbohydrates: Carbohydrate: 9 g   Sugar: 7 g

Citric Acid: 1080 mg

Minerals: Calcium: 9 mg Magnesium: 7 mg Potassium: 128 mg   Phosphorus: 15 mg

Vitamins: Vitamin C: 24 mg

Health Benefits:

The major varieties of grapefruit include Pink, Ruby Red, Star Ruby, Thompson, and White Marsh. Owing to several bioactive phytochemicals, such as flavonoids, carotenoids, coumarins, and organic acids, grapefruit possesses several health-promoting properties such as anti-inflammatory, -cancer, and -obesity effects (Hung et al., 2017).

Blackberry

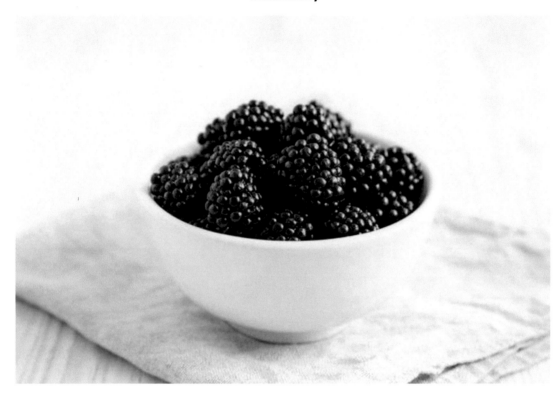

Source Of:

Carbohydrates: Carbohydrate: 9 g   Sugar: 4 g

Minerals: Calcium: 29 mg Magnesium: 20 mg Potassium: 162 mg   Phosphorus: 22mg

Vitamins: Vitamin C: 21 mg

Health Benefits:

Several investigations have focused on the health benefits of consumption of red–black fruit, claiming these as natural sources of bioactive compounds with highly promising antioxidant and anti-inflammatory characteristics. Furthermore, the consumption of red–black berries bring a positive impact on several chronic conditions, such as obesity, diabetes, cancer, cardiovascular and neurodegenerative diseases" (Costa, et. al., 2013).

Lemon

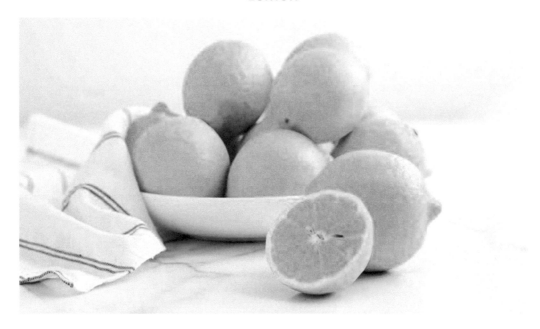

Source Of:

Carbohydrates: Carbohydrate: 9 g   Sugar: 2 g

Minerals: Calcium: 26 mg Magnesium: 8 mg Potassium: 138 mg   Phosphorus: 16 mg

Vitamins: Vitamin C: 53 mg

Health Benefits:

Lemon has many qualities, such as antimicrobial, antifungal, anti-inflammatory, anti-cancer, depurative, antiscorbutic. By drinking one half-cup of lemon juice per day, citrate levels in the urine increase. In tests, lemon juice showed that this could protect the kidney from calcium stones. Soothe a sore throat- Honey mixing with lemon juice can help alleviate and discomfort to treat nasty sore throat. When it comes to bites of insects or poison ivy, rubbing lemon juice on the area will soothe the skin. Anti-inflammatory and anesthetic properties are seen in lemon juice. Studies have supported the citrus liminoids show anticancer activity, compounds that protect cells from damage which is the formation of cancer cells. Drinking a lemon juice mixture can help bring your fever down faster. When body temperature goes up. While lemons may seem quite acidic, lemon is good source of an alkaline food that can help balance pH of body ((Jana et. al., 2020).

Lime

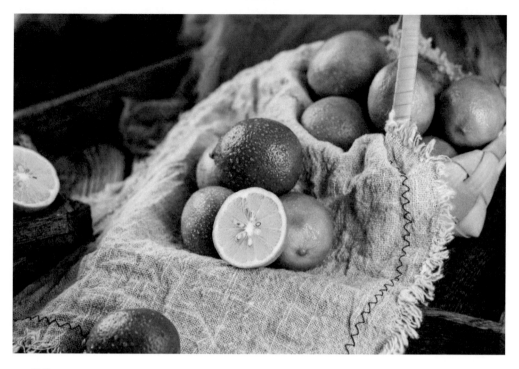

Source Of:

Carbohydrates: Carbohydrate: 8 g   Sugar: 1 g

Minerals: Calcium: 14 mg Magnesium: 8 mg Potassium: 117 mg   Phosphorus: 14mg

Vitamins: Vitamin C: 30 mg

Health Benefits:

Weight loss, skin care, healthy nutrition, constipation relief, eye care and treatment of scurvy, piles, peptic ulcer, respiratory disorders, gout, gums, urinary disorders, etc. are the health benefits of lime. If ingested orally or applied externally, lime juice and its oil are very beneficial to the skin. Owing to the presence of a significant amount of vitamin C and flavonoids, both of which are class 1 anti-oxidants, anti-biotics and disinfectants, it rejuvenates the skin, keeps it bright, protects it from infections. When applied externally to the skin, its acids clean off the dead cells, cure dandruff, rashes, bruises, etc., and if its juice or oil is mixed with your bathing water, give you a soothing bath. Lime has an enticing fragrance that waters the mouth and thus facilitates primary digestion (even before you taste it, the digestive saliva fills your mouth). Then the acids that are in it do the rest (Jana et. al., 2020).

Plum

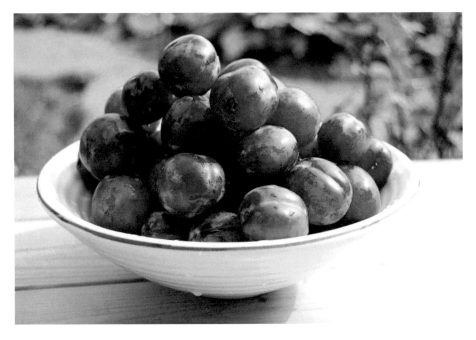

Carbohydrates: Carbohydrate: 11 g   Sugar: 9 g

Minerals: Calcium: 6 mg Magnesium: 7 mg Potassium: 157 mg   Phosphorus: 16 mg

Vitamins: Vitamin C: 30 mg

Health Benefits:

Plums regulates the functioning of the digestive system and thereby relieve constipation conditions due to the presence of dietary fiber, and sorbitol. . Fresh plums, like yellow Mirabelle have moderate vitamin A and beta carotene content. Natural fruit's vitamin A protect from lung and oral cancer. Plums have significant amount of health promoting carotenoids such as lutein, cryptoxanthin and zeaxanthin. These compounds are one kind of scavengers against aging and disease-causing oxygen-derived free radicals and reactive oxygen species. Zeaxanthin provides antioxidant and protective UV light-filtering functions. Plums are rich source of potassium, fluoride and iron. Potassium as an important component of cell and body fluids, helps in controlling heart rate and blood pressure. In addition, the plums are moderate sources in vitamin B-complex groups such as niacin, vitamin B-6 and pantothenic acid and these vitamins help the body metabolize proteins, carbohydrates and fats. Plums also provide about 5% RDA levels of vitamin K. Vitamin K is important for clotting factors function in the blood as well as in bone metabolism and help reduce Alzheimer's disease in the elderly (Birwal et. al., 2017).

Mango

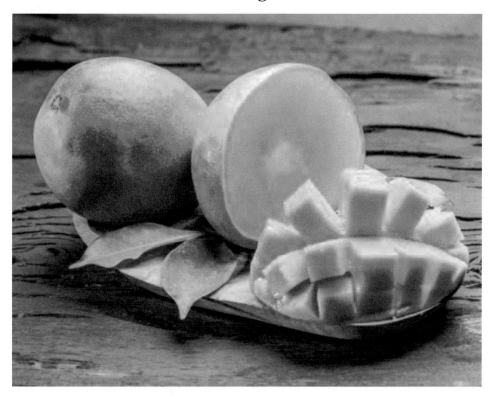

Source of:

Carbohydrates: Carbohydrate: 15 g   Sugar: 13 g

Minerals: Calcium: 11 mg Magnesium: 10 mg Potassium: 168 mg   Phosphorus: 14 mg

Vitamins: Vitamin C: 36 mg

Mango is rich in polyphenols including gallotannins and gallic acid, among others. The bioavailability of mango polyphenols, especially polymeric gallotannins, is largely dependent on the intestinal microbiota, where the generation of absorbable metabolites depends on microbial enzymes. Mango polyphenols can favorably modulate bacteria associated with the production of bioactive gallotannin metabolites including *Lactobacillus plantarum*, resulting in intestinal health benefits. In several studies, the prebiotic effects of mango polyphenols and dietary fiber, their potential contribution to lower intestinal inflammation and promotion of intestinal integrity have been demonstrated. Additionally, polyphenols occurring in mango have some potential to interact with intestinal and less likely with hepatic enzymes or transporter systems (Kim et. al., 2021).

Papaya

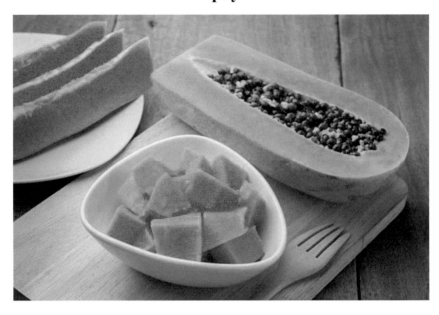

Source of:

Carbohydrates: Carbohydrate: 10 g   Sugar: 7 g

Minerals: Calcium: 20 mg Magnesium: 21 mg Potassium: 182 mg   Phosphorus: 10 mg

Vitamins: Vitamin C: 60 mg

Health Benefits:

Papayas are rich sources of antioxidant nutrients such as carotenes, vitamin C and flavonoids; the B vitamins, folate and pantothenic acid; and the minerals, potassium and magnesium; and fiber. Together, these nutrients promote the health of the cardiovascular system and also provide protection against colon cancer. In addition, papaya contains the digestive enzyme, papain, which is used like bromelain, a similar enzyme found in pineapple, to treat sports injuries, other causes of trauma, and allergies. Papaya's may be very helpful for the prevention of atherosclerosis and diabetic heart disease. Papayas are an excellent source of vitamin C as well as a good source of vitamin E and vitamin A (through their concentration of pro-vitamin A carotenoid phyto nutrients), three very powerful antioxidants. These nutrients help prevent the oxidation of cholesterol. Only when cholesterol becomes oxidized it is able to stick to and build up in blood vessel walls, forming dangerous plaques that can eventually cause heart attacks or strokes (Rahman, 2013).

Apricot

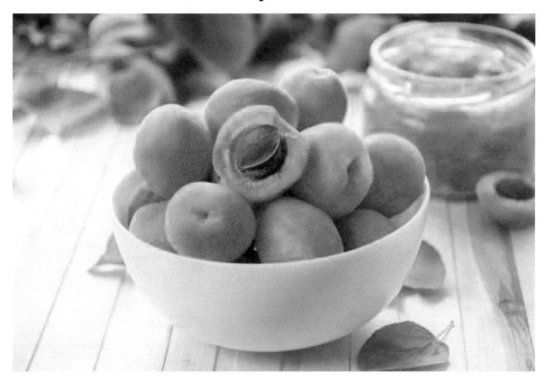

Source of:

Carbohydrates: Carbohydrate: 11 g   Sugar: 9 g

Minerals: Calcium: 13 mg Magnesium: 10 mg Potassium: 259 mg   Phosphorus: 23mg

Vitamins: Vitamin C: 10 mg

Health Benefits:

The scientific evidence reviewed regarding apricot's nutritional and functional attributes reveals that it is a rich source of nutrients and biologically active compounds like polyphenols, carotenoids and vitamins. These substances have crucial roles in disease prevention and health maintenance. The effectiveness of apricot against stomach inflammations, hepatic disorder, tumor formation and chronic heart disease prove it as a functional food (Ali et. al, 2015).

Pomegranate

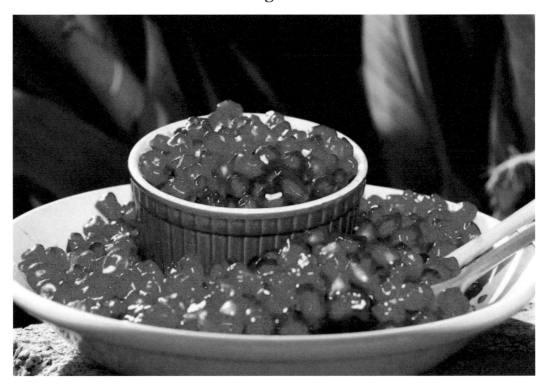

Source Of:

Carbohydrates: Carbohydrate: 18 g   Sugar: 13 g Fiber: 14 g

Minerals: Calcium: 10 mg Magnesium: 12 mg Potassium: 236 mg   Phosphorus: 36 mg

Vitamins: Vitamin C: 10 mg

Oxidative stress is the major contributor of Cardio Vascular Disease (CVD), and inflammation its main manifestation. Reduction of the prevalence of CVD by fruit and vegetable consumption has been well established in several epidemiological studies. In the same way pomegranate intake has shown a high potential in the management of cardio vascular disease (Mena et. al., 2011).

Asparagus

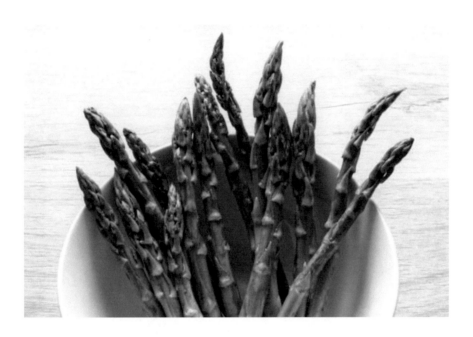

Source of:

Carbohydrates: Carbohydrate: 4 g   Sugar: 1 g Fiber: 2 g

Minerals: Calcium: 23 mg Magnesium: 14 mg Potassium: 224 mg   Phosphorus: 54 mg

Vitamins: Vitamin C: 7 mg

Health Benefits:

Now-a-days, there is an increasing scientific interest in studying the health benefits of asparagus not only for their nutritional properties, but also for their richness in bioactive compounds such as phenols, flavonoids, saponins, bioactive fiber, and sterols. One of the main functions that have been attributed to asparagus saponins for years is its hypolipidemic effect because diets rich in saponins have been shown to lower cholesterol levels, improving the lipid profile. Moreover, it has been shown that the presence of steroidal saponins in the asparagus is able to improve the lipid profile by decreasing the levels of total cholesterol, LDL and triglycerides. Numerous studies have shown the cytotoxic and antitumor properties of steroidal saponins present in asparagus edible part (Hamdi et. al., 2018).

Beet

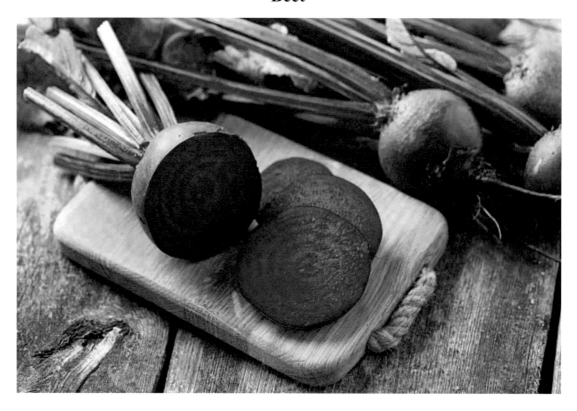

Source of:

Carbohydrates: Carbohydrate: 9 g   Sugar: 6 g Fiber: 2 g

Minerals: Calcium: 16 mg Magnesium: 23 mg Potassium: 325 mg   Phosphorus: 40 mg

Vitamins: Vitamin C: 7 mg

Health Benefits:

Red beetroots are a great source of unique bioactive components called betalains and are rich in polyphenols, antioxidants, vitamins, carotenoids, flavonoids, minerals, and ascorbic acids. Clinical research showed that a dietary intake of nitrate (NO3 −) that is found in beets and from certain vegetables supplies a physiological substrate as the production of nitric oxide (NO), that provide cardiovascular health by reducing blood pressure" (Akan et. al. 2021).

Broccoli

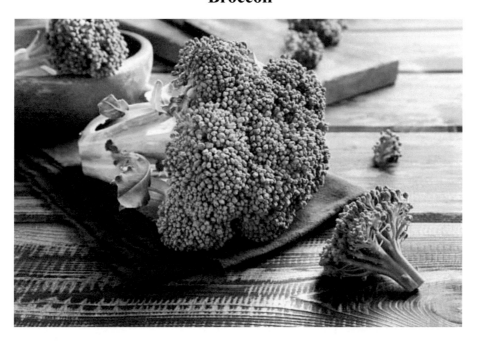

Source of:

Carbohydrates: Carbohydrate: 6 g   Sugar: 1 g Fiber: 2 g

Minerals: Calcium: 47 mg Magnesium: 21 mg Potassium: 316 mg   Phosphorus: 66 mg

Vitamins: Vitamin C: 89 mg

Health Benefits:

Mahn (2012), states "the intake of this vegetable results in an improvement of the general health status, mainly due to its antioxidant (Borowski et al., 2008) and anticarcinogenic properties (Jeffery and Araya, 2009). These beneficial effects are exerted by the action of some bioactive compounds present in broccoli that positively affect mainly the immune system and the antioxidant defense of the individuals that consume it. Among these compounds, glucosinolates, sulforaphane, polyphenols and minerals such as selenium are of major interest (Moreno et al., 2006). Besides, broccoli, as most vegetables, is a good source of minerals, such as calcium, magnesium, phosphorus, potassium and sodium, which can be affected in different ways by domestic or technological processing (Kmiecik et al., 2007).

Brussel Sprouts

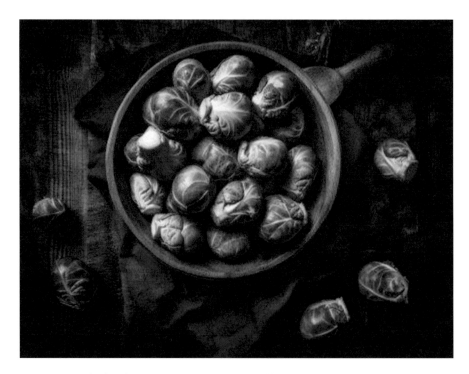

Carbohydrates: Carbohydrate: 9 g   Sugar: 2 g Fiber: 3 g

Minerals: Calcium: 47 mg Iron: 1mg

Vitamins: Vitamin A: 882 IU Vitamin C: 84 mg

Health Benefits:

Evidence from human studies that enzyme systems in our cells required for detoxification of cancer-causing substances can be activated by compounds made from glucosinolates found in Brussel sprouts. Brussel sprouts contain carotenoids, vitamin C, fiber, and flavonoids. Also, they have antibacterial, fungicide and anticancer effect. Clarke et al. examined the anticancer effect of sulforaphane in case of broccoli, cabbage, Brussels sprouts and cauliflower. It was established that sulforaphane occurs in an especially high concentration in the broccoli and broccoli sprout and due to its high isothiocyanate content reduces the risk of cancer including intestine and prostate cancer (Awulachew, 2022).

Cabbage

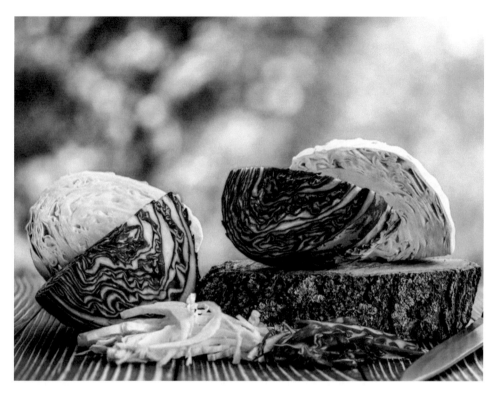

Source of:

Carbohydrates: Carbohydrate: 5 g   Sugar: 3 g Fiber: 2 g

Minerals: Calcium: 40 mg Magnesium: 12 mg Potassium: 170 mg   Phosphorus: 26 mg

Vitamins: Vitamin C: 36 mg

Health Benefits:

Podsędek, and Combs states "Associated with vitamin C, carotenoids and tocopherols (vitamin E analogs) are compounds with demonstrated antioxidant activity to be part of the health benefits of white cabbage (Podsędek, 2007). In addition to antioxidant properties, vitamin A precursors like α-carotene and β-carotene 158 are needed for healthy skin, bones, gastrointestinal and respiratory systems. While vitamin E which has neurological functions, regulates enzyme activity and gene expression, vitamin C has a role to play in enhancing the immune system (Alexandra, et.al. 2020).

Carrots

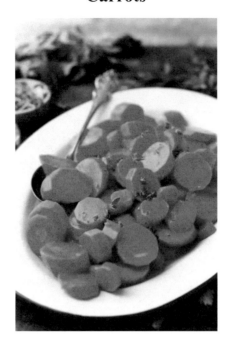

Source of:

Carbohydrates: Carbohydrate: 9 g   Sugar: 4 g Fiber: 2 g

Minerals: Calcium: 33 mg Magnesium: 12 mg Potassium: 320 mg   Phosphorus: 35 mg

Vitamins: Vitamin C: 5 mg

Health Benefits:

Carrots, like many or colorful vegetables, are high in antioxidants. Carrots' biological & rapeutic effects may be due to the high concentration of antioxidant carotenoids, particularly -carotene. Antioxidants are found in carrots in form of carotenoids, polyphenols, & vitamins. Carrots offer anti-inflammatory properties. Carrots protect human heart from oxidative damage, plaque development, & harmful cholesterol increase when consumed regularly. This is due to presence of soluble fibers that bind to bile acids. Carrots' antioxidants & phytochemicals may help control blood sugar levels, making m anti-diabetic. To prevent high blood pressure & heart disease, American Heart Association (AHA) recommends eating a fiber-rich diet & boosting potassium while lowering salt consumption. Skin disorders like pimples & acne, rashes, dermatitis, & or skin issues caused by Vitamin A deficiency may be treated with antioxidants included in carrots (Varshney et. al., 2022).

Cauliflower

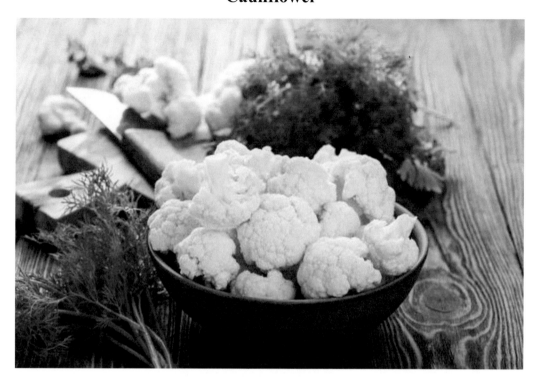

Source of:

Carbohydrates: Carbohydrate: 4 g   Sugar: 1 g Fiber: 2 g

Minerals: Calcium: 22 mg Magnesium: 15 mg Potassium: 299 mg   Phosphorus: 44 mg

Vitamins: Vitamin C: 48 mg

Health Benefits:

Cruciferous vegetables, cauliflower, also serve as a good source of carbohydrates, which ranges from 0.3% to 10%. Calcium, phosphorous, magnesium, sodium and potassium constitute major macro elements and iron, selenium, copper, manganese and zinc are micronutrients found in cruciferous vegetables. The report concluded that small quantities of cruciferous vegetables like cauliflower may offer more protection against risk of cancer as compared to large quantities of mature vegetables (Manchali et al., 2012).

Celery

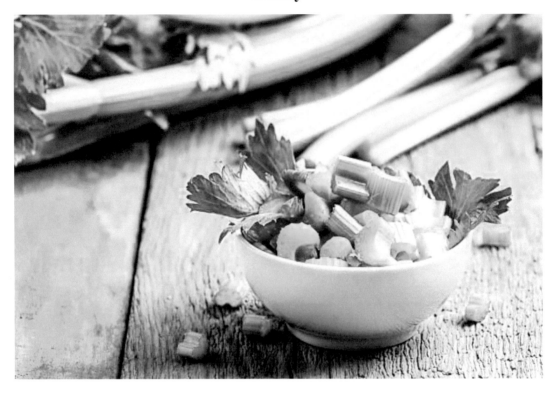

Source of:

Carbohydrates: Carbohydrate: 2 g   Sugar: 1 g Fiber: 1 g

Minerals: Calcium: 40 mg Magnesium: 11 mg Potassium: 260 mg   Phosphorus: 24 mg

Vitamins: Vitamin C: 3 mg

Health Benefits:

Different parts of celery contain fatty acids, volatile essential oils, vitamins and minerals such as potassium, magnesium and calcium along with chlorophyll, silica, β-carotene, fibers, sodium and folic acid. Celery has anti-inflammatory, antimicrobial, anti-fungal, anti-bacterial, anti-virus, anti-cancer, anti-spasmodic, gastro-intestinal and anti-oxidant potentials properties. It is also known as a rich source of vitamin C and various other minerals (Khalil et. al., 2015).

Cucumber

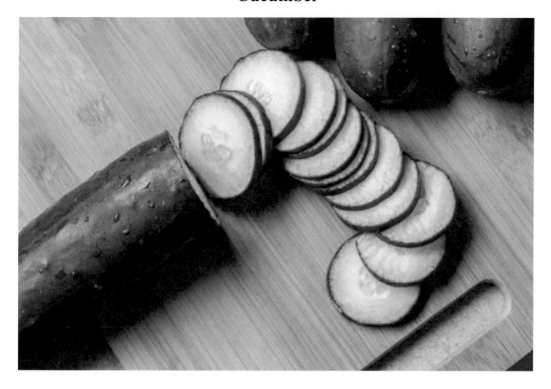

Carbohydrates: Carbohydrate: 3 g   Sugar: 1 g Fiber: 0.5 g

Minerals: Calcium: 16 mg Magnesium: 13 mg Potassium: 147 mg   Phosphorus: 24 mg

Vitamins: Vitamin C: 2 mg

Health Benefits:

It is widely used as medicine in traditional Indian medical practices and very much liked as vegetable. Cucumber fruit consists more than ninety percentage of water, offers superior hydration, and is very low in calories as a food. Its flavor and texture have made it essential as a fresh addition to salads and in processed forms such as pickles and relishes. It exhibits various medicinal properties like antimicrobial activity, glycemic lowering ability, antioxidant ability, etc., and is traditionally used in various treatments. It is believed that its regular intake or application on skin helps in reducing the aging effect, boosting metabolism, and improving immunity (Sharma. et. al., 2020).

Eggplant

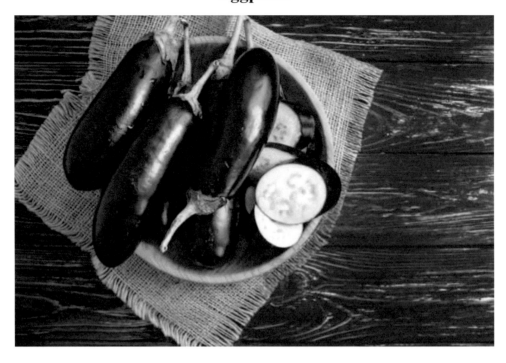

Carbohydrates: Carbohydrate: 5 g   Sugar: 3 g Fiber: 3 g

Minerals: Calcium: 9 mg Magnesium: 14 mg Potassium: 229 mg   Phosphorus: 24 mg

Vitamins: Vitamin C: 2 mg

Health Benefits:

Various research shows that the eggplant extracts have superb healing effects on different disorders like burns, warts, inflammatory infections, gastritis, stomatitis and arthritis. Eggplant is producing a widespread choice of various secondary metabolites along with some other compounds such as glycol-alkaloids, antioxidant compounds, and vitamins which carried a significant part in keeping   good   health. Casati et al. (2016), states "Eggplants   are   the   rich   source   of anthocyanin compounds, besides their coloring functions. It has been known   that   anthocyanin has significant   role   against diabetes, neuronal problems, cardiovascular disorders, and cancer as well (Naeem & Ugur, 2019).

Garlic

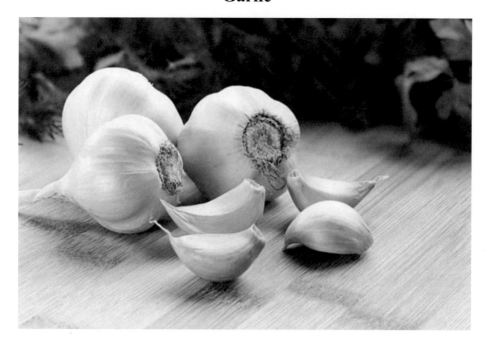

Carbohydrates: Carbohydrate: 33 g   Sugar: 1 g Fiber: 2 g

Minerals: Calcium: 181 mg Magnesium: 25 mg Potassium: 401 mg   Phosphorus: 153 mg

Vitamins: Vitamin C: 31 mg

Health Benefits:

Past decades have seen myriad studies, especially in vitro and in animal models, addressing the protective effect of garlic against cardiovascular disease and cancer. This protection can arise from its diverse biological activities: enhanced antioxidant defense, lowering of blood lipids, inhibition of blood aggregation, enhancement of cancer cell cycle arrest/ apoptosis, inhibition of invasion and/or metastasis, and modulation of drug metabolism and/or the immune response". Numerous studies have demonstrated garlic and its organosulfur compounds to be potent antioxidants by displaying radical-scavenging activity and modulating cellular antioxidant enzyme activity (Tsai et al., 2012).

Ginger

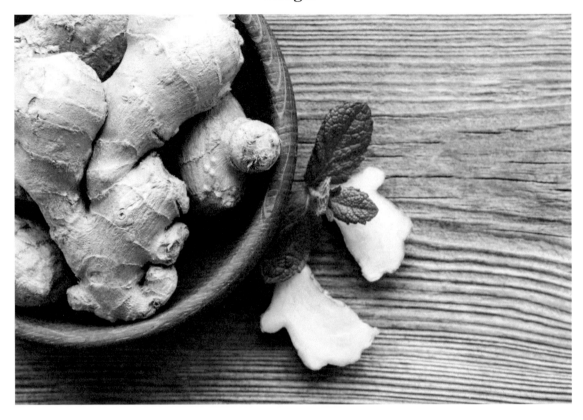

Carbohydrates: Carbohydrate: 17 g   Sugar: 1 g Fiber: 2 g

Minerals: Calcium: 16 mg Magnesium: 43 mg Potassium: 415 mg   Phosphorus: 34 mg

Vitamins: Vitamin C: 5 mg

Health Benefits:

Jiang et al (2006), states, it also has anti-inflammatory properties, and these properties are beneficial in controlling the process of aging. Also, it is recommended for sore throat and vomiting. Moreover, it has antimicrobial potential as well which can help in treating infectious diseases and helminthiasis Butt, et al., (2011).

Lettuce

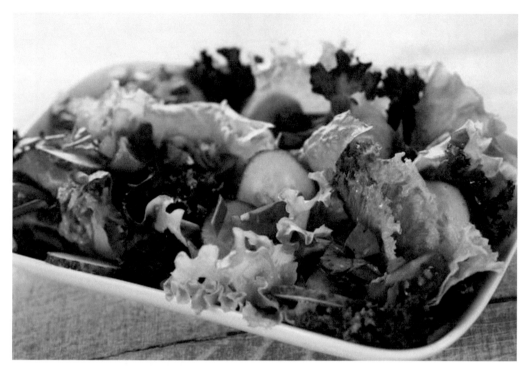

Carbohydrates: Carbohydrate: 2 g   Sugar: 3 g Fiber: 1 g

Minerals: Calcium: 36 mg Magnesium: 13 mg Potassium: 194 mg   Phosphorus: 29 mg

Vitamins: Vitamin C: 9 mg

Health Benefits:

Lettuce contains around 95% water, compared to spinach's approximately 91%. This means that the nutrients found in lettuce are distributed across a much greater volume of plant tissue because the nutrients are, in effect, diluted by the water content. Lettuce vitamin contents depend on the type of lettuce and growing conditions, but in general, many lettuces supply a significant amount of Vitamin A and Vitamin K to human diets. According to Harsha and Kim "Ultraviolet radiation and temperature are two other environmental factors that have a significant influence on lettuce nutrition, particularly Vitamin A and antioxidants. Together, these compounds have been demonstrated to reduce harmful free radicals in the body (Harsha et al. 2013), leading to reductions in cholesterol and diabetes markers in mice studies, as well as correlations to reduced incidences in colorectal and lung cancer in humans (Murray et al., 2021).

Onion

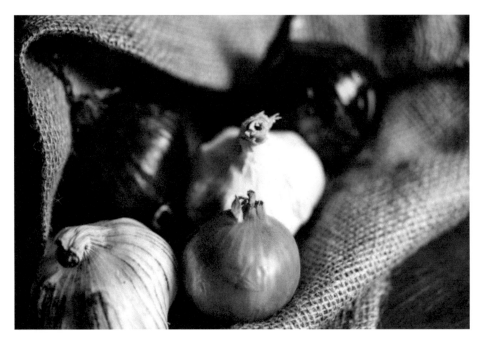

Carbohydrates: Carbohydrate: 9 g   Sugar: 4 g Fiber: 1 g

Minerals: Calcium: 23 mg Magnesium: 10 mg Potassium: 146 mg   Phosphorus: 29 mg

Vitamins: Vitamin C: 7 mg

Health Benefits:

Although rarely used specifically as a medicinal herb, the onion has a wide range of beneficial actions on the body and when eaten (especially raw) on a regular basis will promote the general health of the body. The bulb is anthelmintic, anti-inflammatory, antiseptic, antispasmodic, carminative, diuretic, expectorant, febrifuge, hypoglycaemic, hypotensive, lithontripic, stomachic and tonic. When used regularly in the diet it offsets tendencies towards angina, arteriosclerosis and heart attack. This is used particularly in the treatment of people whose symptoms include running eyes and nose. The onion's ability to relieve congestions especially in the lungs and bronchial tract, is hard to believe until you have actually witnessed the results. The drawing of infection, congestion and colds out of the ear is also remarkable. The onion will relieve stomach upset and other gastrointestinal disorders and it will also strengthen the appetite. The onion also may be of benefit in cardiovascular disease, as it possesses hypolipidemic effects and has antiplatelet actions, retarding thrombosis (Kumar et al., 2010).

Bell Pepper

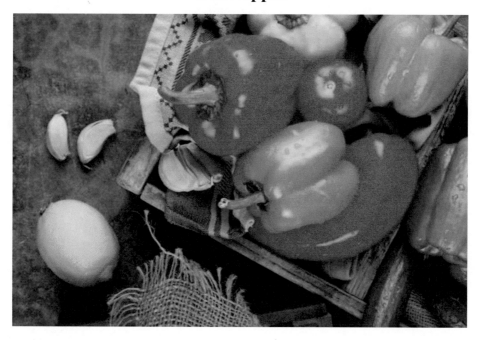

Carbohydrates: Carbohydrate: 6 g   Sugar: 4 g Fiber: 2 g

Minerals: Calcium: 7 mg Magnesium: 12 mg Potassium: 211mg   Phosphorus: 26 mg

Vitamins: Vitamin C: 128 mg

Health Benefits:

Bell Pepper is good source of vitamin C. The benefits resulting from the use of natural products rich in bioactive substances has promoted the growing interest of food industries. Among the antioxidant phytochemicals, polyphenols deserve a special mention due to their free radical scavenging properties. Antioxidant compounds and their antioxidant activity in 4 different colored (green, yellow, orange, and red) are in sweet bell peppers. (GMF, 2008), states "Bell peppers offer a number of nutritional values. They are excellent sources of vitamin C and vitamin A. They also are a source of vitamin B6, folic acid, beta-carotene, and fiber. Red peppers also contain lycopene, believed important for reducing risk of certain cancers (Nadeem et al., 2011).

Spinach

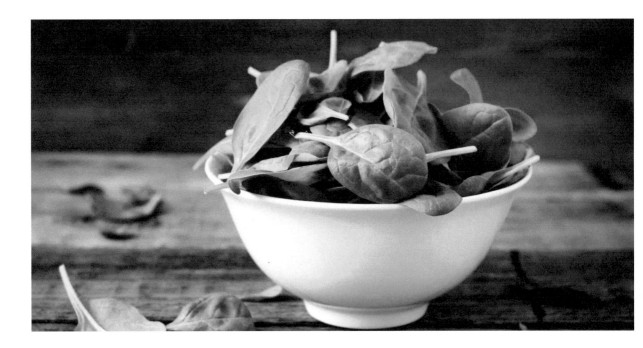

Carbohydrates: Carbohydrate: 3 g   Fiber: 2 g

Minerals: Calcium: 99 mg Iron: 2 mg Magnesium: 79 mg Potassium: 558 mg   Phosphorus: 49 mg

Vitamins: Vitamin C: 28 mg

Health Benefits:

Spinach flavonoids have shown to possess anticancer, antioxidant, α-amylase, bile acid binding and anti-inflammatory activities. Polyphenols that are in spinach possess various health benefits such as anticancer, anti-inflammatory, cardiovascular health, scavenging of free radicals, and also antimicrobial activities. Several studies demonstrated that the consumption of fruits and vegetables are beneficial to human health by reducing the risk of chronic diseases (22). Spinach is a well-known leafy vegetable rich in several health promoting compounds such as carotenoids, flavonoids, ascorbic acid, chlorophyll, vitamin E and nitrate (Singh et al., 2018).

Tomatoes

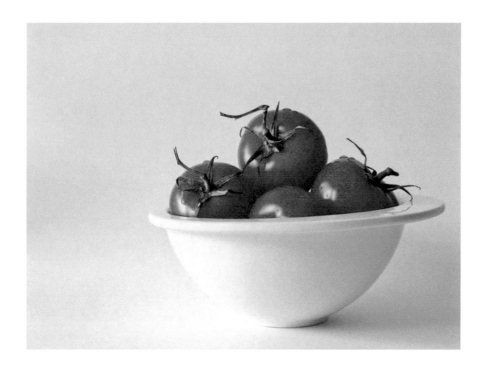

Carbohydrates: Carbohydrate: 4 g   Sugar: 2 g Fiber: g

Minerals: Calcium: 11 mg Magnesium: 9 mg Potassium: 218 mg   Phosphorus: 28 mg

Vitamins: Vitamin C: 22 mg

Studies conducted by Harvard researchers have discovered that men who consumed 10 servings of tomatoes a week, or the equivalent to 10 slices of pizza, can cut the risk of developing prostate cancer by a formidable 45 percent. Italian researchers have found that those who consume more than 7 servings of raw tomatoes lower the risk of developing rectal colon or stomach cancers by 60 percent. Italian researchers have found that those who consume more than 7 servings of raw tomatoes lower the risk of developing rectal colon or stomach cancers by 60 percent. Lastly, new research is beginning to indicate that tomatoes may be used to help prevent lung cancer (Kumar et al.,2012).

Yellow Squash

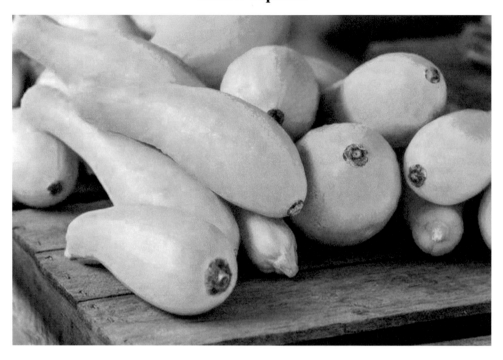

Carbohydrates: Carbohydrate: 3 g   Sugar: 2 g Fiber: 1 g

Minerals: Calcium: 16 mg Magnesium: 18 mg Potassium: 261 mg   Phosphorus: 38 mg

Vitamins: Vitamin C: 17 mg

Health Benefits:

Squash has health benefits such as anti-diabetic antifungal, antibacterial and antiinflammation. Squash is a good source of pro-vitamin A and have antioxidant activity. Several reports stated that many minerals are considered to be essential in nutrition and they are important constituents of bones, teeth, tissues, muscles, blood and nerve cells. Generally, the minerals help in the maintenance of acid-base balance, the response of nerves to physiological stimulation and blood clotting. A study revealed that the Squash has high contents of K and Na. Therefore, Squash is very important in the diet for prevention of high blood pressure" (Hashash et al.,2017).

Zucchini

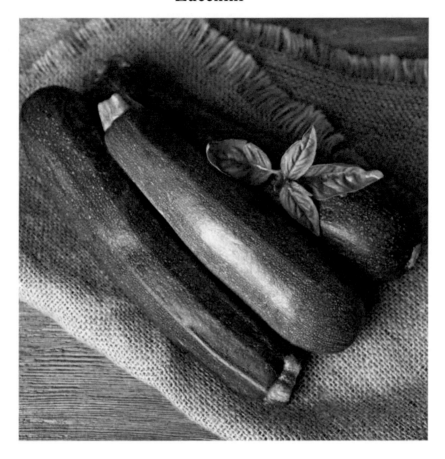

Carbohydrates: Carbohydrate: 3 g   Sugar: 2 g Fiber: 1 g

Minerals: Calcium: 16 mg Magnesium: 18 mg Potassium: 261 mg   Phosphorus: 38 mg

Vitamins: Vitamin C: 17 mg

Health Benefits:

Zucchini is one of the lowest caloric content vegetables (14 kcal/100 g) and has the highest water content (96.5%). Its consumption covers the needs of vitamins and minerals, especially vitamin C and potassium, vitamin C being the most significant. The presence of mucilage gives it emollient properties on the digestive system and as an easy-to-digest food, it is suitable for those with digestive problems (Tejada et al., 2020).

Beans and Legumes

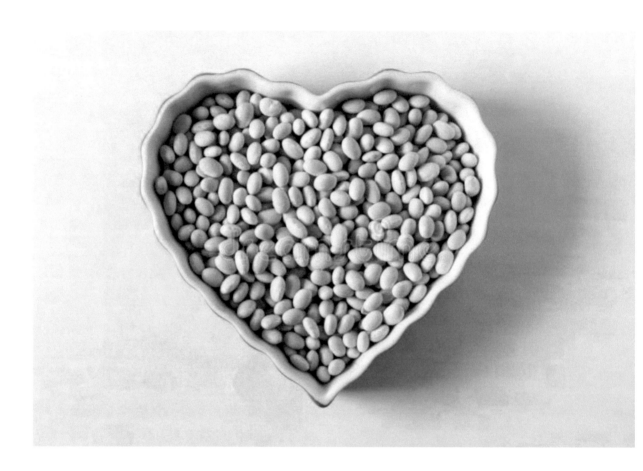

Navy Beans

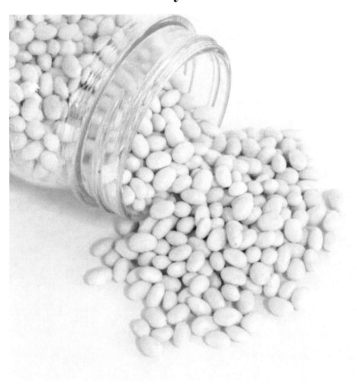

Carbohydrates:

Protein: 8 gr **Carbohydrates:** Carbohydrate: 26 g   Sugar: 0 g Fiber: 2 g

Minerals: Calcium: 69 mg Magnesium: 53 mg Potassium: 389 mg   Phosphorus: 144 mg Iron: 2 mg Zinc: 1 mg

Navy beans are white in color, and were used in the U.S. Navy diet during the 19th century; hence, their name. They are small-sized, white-skinned, oval-shaped beans. Navy bean-containing diets exerted beneficial effects during experimental colitis by reducing inflammatory biomarkers both locally and systemically. Emerging evidence supports the efficacy of navy beans in regulating serum cholesterol and lipid profiles, and inhibiting the incidence and recurrence of adenomatous polyps or precancerous growths, thereby preventing colorectal cancer. Navy bean-containing diets exerted beneficial effects during experimental colitis by reducing inflammatory biomarkers both locally and systemically (Ganesan et al., 2017).

Lentils

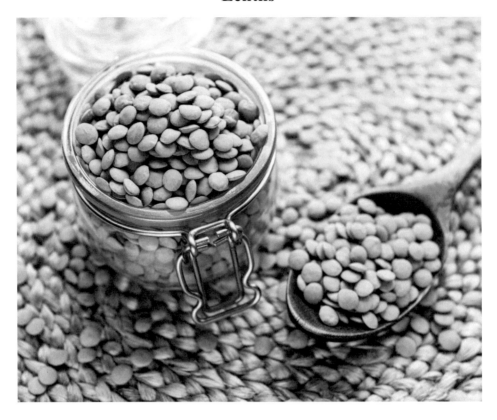

Carbohydrates: Carbohydrate: 6 3 g   Sugar: 1 g Fiber: 2 g

Minerals: Calcium: 62 mg Iron: 7mg Magnesium: 107 mg Potassium: 949 mg   Phosphorus: 374 mg Zinc: 3 mg

The health benefits have been described for lentils such as anticarcinogenic, blood pressure-lowering, hypocholesterolemic and glycemic load lowering effects" (Lentils are a significant dietary source of a plethora of vitamins including folate, thiamin (B1) and riboflavin (B2) [12]. Other water-soluble vitamins have also been reported in lentils as follows: niacin; pantothenic acid and pyridoxine. In addition, vitamin E. Lentils contain considerably high amount of the pivotal folic acid, which is expected to be involved in the cancer preventive effect of lentils' (Faris, 2013).

References

Akan, S., Tuna Gunes, N., & Erkan, M. (2021). Red beetroot: Health benefits, production techniques, and quality maintaining for food industry. *Journal of Food Processing and Preservation, 45*(10), e15781. https://www.researchgate.net/profile/Selen-Akan/publication/353467831_Red_Beetroot_Health_benefits_production_techniques_and_quality_maintaining_for_food_industry/links/610b91170c2bfa282a23880b/Red-Beetroot-Health-benefits-production-techniques-and-quality-maintaining-for-food-industry.pdf

Alexandra, Ş. I. M., & Andreea Daniela, O. N. A. (2020). Cabbage (Brassica oleracea l.). Overview of the health benefits and therapeutical uses. *Hop. and Medicinal Plants, Year,* 1-2.https://odontoanamaria.com/artigos/repolho01.pdf

Ali, S., Masud, T., Abbasi, K. S., Mahmood, T., & Hussain, A. (2015). Apricot: nutritional potentials and health benefits-a review. *Annals: Food Science & Technology, 16*(1). https://afst.valahia.ro/wp-content/uploads/2022/09/s02_w06_full_2015.pdf

Awulachew, M. T. (2022). A Review to Nutritional and Health Aspect of Sprouted Food. *Int. J. Food Sci. Nutr. Diet, 10*(7), 564-568.https://www.researchgate.net/profile/Melaku-Awulachew/publication/357714401_A_Review_to_Nutritional_and_Health_Aspect_of_Sprouted_Food/links/61dc4e44034dda1b9eea72f8/A-Review-to-Nutritional-and-Health-Aspect-of-Sprouted-Food.pdf

Ayad, A. A., Williams, L. L., Gad El-Rab, D. A., Ayivi, R., Colleran, H. L., Aljaloud, S., & Ibrahim, S. A. (2020). A review of the chemical composition, nutritional and health benefits of dates for their potential use in energy nutrition bars for athletes. *Cogent Food & Agriculture, 6*(1), 1809309. https://www.tandfonline.com/doi/full/10.1080/23311932.2020.1809309

Bento, C., Goncalves, A. C., Silva, B., & Silva, L. R. (2022). Peach (Prunus persica): Phytochemicals and health benefits. *Food Reviews International, 38*(8), 1703-1734. https://www.tandfonline.com/doi/abs/10.1080/87559129.2020.1837861

Birwal, P., Deshmukh, G., Saurabh, S. P., & Pragati, S. (2017). Plums: a brief introduction. *Journal of Food, Nutrition and Population Health, 1*(1), 1-5. https://www.researchgate.net/profile/Saurabh-Patel-12/publication/316514807_Plums_A_Brief_Introduction/links/5901d66baca2725bd721b806/Plums-A-Brief-Introduction.pdf

Boyer, J., & Liu, R. H. (2004). Apple phytochemicals and their health benefits. *Nutrition journal*, *3*, 1-15. https://link.springer.com/article/10.1186/1475-2891-3-5

Butt, M. S., & Sultan, M. T. (2011). Ginger and its health claims: molecular aspects. *Critical reviews in food science and nutrition*, *51*(5), 383-393.https://web.archive.org/web/20190308213456id_/http://pdfs.semanticscholar.org/f9b4/2ea0627c8a2dfa8bfbf92b69c220192e2151.pdf

Daub, M. R. Health Benefits Of Grapes. https://my.klarity.health/health-benefits-of-grapes/

Costa, A. G. V., Garcia-Diaz, D. F., Jimenez, P., & Silva, P. I. (2013). Bioactive compounds and health benefits of exotic tropical red–black berries. *Journal of functional foods*, *5*(2), 539-549. https://www.sciencedirect.com/science/article/abs/pii/S1756464613000479

Duarte, P. F., Chaves, M. A., Borges, C. D., & Mendonça, C. R. B. (2016). Avocado: characteristics, health benefits and uses. *Ciência rural*, *46*, 747-754. https://www.scielo.br/j/cr/a/VqMdKHmY4y5zHgtJKjc98nS/?lang=en

Faris, M. E. A. I. E., Takruri, H. R., & Issa, A. Y. (2013). Role of lentils (Lens culinaris L.) in human health and nutrition: a review. *Mediterranean Journal of Nutrition and Metabolism*, *6*(1), 3-16.

Giampieri, F., Tulipani, S., Alvarez-Suarez, J. M., Quiles, J. L., Mezzetti, B., & Battino, M. (2012). The strawberry: Composition, nutritional quality, and impact on human health. *Nutrition*, *28*(1), 9-19. https://www.sciencedirect.com/science/article/abs/pii/S0899900711003066

Hamdi, A., Jiménez Araujo, A., Rodríguez-Arcos, R., Jaramillo Carmona, S. M., Lachaal, M., Bouraoui, N. K., & Guillén Bejarano, R. (2018). Asparagus saponins: chemical characterization, bioavailability and intervention in human health. https://digital.csic.es/bitstream/10261/176566/1/NFSIJ_2018_V7_555704.pdf

Hashash, M. M., El-Sayed, M. M., Abdel-Hady, A. A., Hady, H. A., & Morsi, E. A. (2017). Nutritional potential, mineral composition and antioxidant activity squash (Curcurbita pepo L.) fruits grown in Egypt. *inflammation*, *9*(10), 11-12. https://www.researchgate.net/profile/Eman-Morsi/publication/321018398_NUTRITIONAL_POTENTIAL_MINERAL_COMPOSITION_AND_ANTIOXIDANT_ACTIVITY_SQUASH_CUCURBITA_PEPO_L_FRUITS_GROWN_IN_EGYPT/links/5a0865140f7e9b68229c96d6/NUTRITIONAL-POTENTIAL-MINERAL-COMPOSITION-AND-ANTIOXIDANT-ACTIVITY-SQUASH-CUCURBITA-PEPO-L-FRUITS-GROWN-IN-EGYPT.pdf

Ganesan, K., & Xu, B. (2017). Polyphenol-rich dry common beans (Phaseolus vulgaris L.) and their health benefits. *International journal of molecular sciences*, *18*(11), 2331. https://www.mdpi.com/1422-0067/18/11/2331

Ismail, H. I., Chan, K. W., Mariod, A. A., & Ismail, M. (2010). Phenolic content and antioxidant activity of cantaloupe (Cucumis melo) methanolic extracts. *Food chemistry*, *119*(2), 643-647.https://www.researchgate.net/profile/Kim-Wei-Chan/publication/223065931_Phenolic_content_and_antioxidant_activity_of_cantaloupe_Cucumis_melo_methanolic_extracts/links/5addd76f458515c60f5f75b4/Phenolic-content-and-antioxidant-activity-of-cantaloupe-Cucumis-melo-methanolic-extracts.pdf

Jana, P., Sureshrao, P. A., & Sahu, R. S. (2020). Medicinal and health benefits of lemon. *Journal of Science and Technology*, *6*, 16-20. https://jst.org.in/admin/uploads/03.-Medicinal-and-Health-Benefits-of-Lemon.pdf

Jayarajan, S., Sharma, R. R., Sethi, S., Saha, S., Sharma, V. K., & Singh, S. (2019). Chemical and nutritional evaluation of major genotypes of nectarine (Prunus persica var nectarina) grown in North-Western Himalayas. *Journal of food science and technology*, *56*, 4266-4273. https://www.ncbi.nlm.nih.gov/pmc/articles/PMC6706499/

Kelley, D. S., Adkins, Y., & Laugero, K. D. (2018). A review of the health benefits of cherries. *Nutrients*, *10*(3), 368. https://www.mdpi.com/2072-6643/10/3/368

Hypocrites (820 BC).

Khalid, W., Ikram, A., Rehan, M., Afzal, F. A., Ambreen, S., Ahmad, M., ... & Sadiq, A. (2021). Chemical composition and health benefits of melon seed: A Review. *PJAR*, *34*, 309-317. https://www.researchgate.net/profile/Waseem-Khalid-4/publication/351109040_Chemical_Composition_and_Health_Benefits_of_Melon_Seed_A_Review/links/6087e6ec881fa114b42e0b88/Chemical-Composition-and-Health-Benefits-of-Melon-Seed-A-Review.pdf

Khalil, A., Nawaz, H., Ghania, J. B., Rehman, R., & Nadeem, F. (2015). Value added products, chemical constituents and medicinal uses of celery (Apium graveolens L.)–A review. *International Journal of Chemical and Biochemical Sciences*, *8*(2015), 40-48. https://iscientific.org/wp-content/uploads/2019/09/6-IJCBS-15-08-06.pdf

Kim, H., Castellon-Chicas, M. J., Arbizu, S., Talcott, S. T., Drury, N. L., Smith, S., &

Kumar, K. S., Paswan, S., & Srivastava, S. (2012). Tomato-a natural medicine and its health benefits. *Journal of Pharmacognosy and Phytochemistry*, *1*(1), 33-43.

https://www.phytojournal.com/archives?year=2012&vol=1&issue=1&ArticleId=5&si=false

Mertens-Talcott, S. U. (2021). Mango (Mangifera indica L.) polyphenols: Anti-inflammatory intestinal microbial health benefits, and associated mechanisms of actions. *Molecules*, *26*(9), 2732. https://www.mdpi.com/1420-3049/26/9/2732

Kumar, K. S., Bhowmik, D., Chiranjib, B., & Tiwari, P. (2010). Allium cepa: A traditional medicinal herb and its health benefits. *Journal of Chemical and Pharmaceutical Research*, *2*(1), 283-291. https://d1wqtxts1xzle7.cloudfront.net/34504139/allium_cepa-libre.pdf?1408664482=&response-content-disposition=inline%3B+filename%3DAvailable_on_line_www_Allium_cepa_A_trad.pdf&Expires=1705700992&Signature=X~hPCi80KEBr0VGWaUiQL~u8aX4s61SNuNbbQ2790A3FO7FhcHZluy-q3b2RDY6jcd~toBwJYQQQaBUQX9e15y0rtZ1FmKerY1kKIRl5CT9UcZREbZRJyKULO62Ft03ptCcEf9QqAHxCjVSTAj1L4GXJJZY4skH1pe01va4rq6pVZZcHP~1XFm9OvLcCBGd-mu8oJWhZxh7OVrvyoRjBRiECfLVQTXP2ugV9GupcKDkZn~z~5hi3IovHbUR0IPrJO6zMp812ZVSmMqGh2dKZD~T80GojCbFgC3bS-Wk06bURfQG~xuw-h9pIHoUOH1M0wZwQ-eqa03uLoRvL8kTW3g__&Key-Pair-Id=APKAJLOHF5GGSLRBV4ZA

Manchali, S., Murthy, K. N. C., & Patil, B. S. (2012). Crucial facts about health benefits of popular cruciferous vegetables. *Journal of functional foods*, *4*(1), 94-106. https://www.sciencedirect.com/science/article/pii/S1756464611000843

Maoto, M. M., Beswa, D., & Jideani, A. I. (2019). Watermelon as a potential fruit snack. *International Journal of food properties*, *22*(1), 355-370. **https://www.tandfonline.com/doi/full/10.1080/10942912.2019.1584212**

Mahn, A., & Reyes, A. (2012). An overview of health-promoting compounds of broccoli (Brassica oleracea var. italica) and the effect of processing. *Food science and technology international*, *18*(6), 503-514. https://d1wqtxts1xzle7.cloudfront.net/52637537/An_overview_of_health-promoting_compound20170416-3556-rhbwef-libre.pdf?1492358278=&response-content-disposition=inline%3B+filename%3DAn_overview_of_health_promoting_compound.pdf&Expires=1705531532&Signature=YV61AlMSrQ9g-qnPZI0cDmoVeQF0fFRAXkglaRXfjgk5NWJRhe19luOP1pNNEAnS6VnqpVg7J-3PLoNF3uM9Bzgsx0rHcVQFzelS2ghZ-l3-VyWkSGLkfNz6kVv69uZiRr8O5keb~7suALH2aziRH~GWM-

8UzoGCV~3~zcoYMVyLiNftR2-Q-
d0GUhU5Q~91d8oifKRPZ4zGPVf62JbqmBUyMwXA0xEzuqx7LytfnWNhgzG1v1hvp
o9SDHxvQT5q3VwjHlM4SwGgq-
c5IRcN1hh6FkBjTe~zLWE~IdRYHnXoOT6tXiOq0tJCGF3xAKPgZMIfdRWxtCRoukL
eyHNlPA__&Key-Pair-Id=APKAJLOHF5GGSLRBV4ZA

Mena, P., Gironés-Vilaplana, A., Moreno, D. A., & García-Viguera, C. (2011).
Pomegranate fruit for health promotion: Myths and realities. *Funct Plant Sci
Biotechnol*, *5*, 33-42.
http://www.globalsciencebooks.info/Online/GSBOnline/images/2011/FPSB_5(SI2)/FPS
B_5(SI2)33-42o.pdf

Mohsin, A., Jabeen, A., Majid, D., Allai, F. M., Dar, A. H., Gulzar, B., & Makroo, H. A.
(2020). Pineapple. *Antioxidants in fruits: Properties and health benefits*, 379-396.
https://link.springer.com/chapter/10.1007/978-981-15-7285-2_19

Muhammad, E. (1972). How to eat to live.

Murray, J. J., Basset, G., & Sandoya, G. (2021). Nutritional Benefits of Lettuce
Consumed at Recommended Portion Sizes. *Edis*, *3*, 1-
8.https://www.researchgate.net/profile/Jesse-Murray-
3/publication/353062924_Nutritional_Benefits_of_Lettuce_Consumed_at_Recommende
d_Portion_Sizes/links/60ec56a4fb568a7098a38440/Nutritional-Benefits-of-Lettuce-
Consumed-at-Recommended-Portion-Sizes.pdf

Nadeem, M., Anjum, F. M., Khan, M. R., Saeed, M., & Riaz, A. (2011). Antioxidant
potential of bell pepper (Capsicum annum L.)-A review. *Pakistan Journal of Food
Science*, *21*(1-4), 45-
51.https://d1wqtxts1xzle7.cloudfront.net/50222750/Antioxidant_Potential_of_Bell_Pepp
er_Ca20161109-8360-h3m2nd-libre.pdf?1478764896=&response-content-
disposition=inline%3B+filename%3DAntioxidant_Potential_of_Bell_Pepper_Cap.pdf&
Expires=1705701486&Signature=IolaxNZ-
gHLyCg8bSdDMscZIjf18nLXeZByLNXRw70N9jVJAkdG~S1DZVMi7g09G318NHGc
bNud-~uAFXBTqstv~cLOXn~rstOfFmoyAOeX-~VObYBG5v-KsND524gip9iGX5W-
nSqhKRxMPMapzs3mEn3qTT7YvAiQZJ58GiviOngRwWRMAVpSwDaRKDfkdUoWc
DcDGoqNs6M6VKteDD92Sc2J8FGbF~RJpZ9sOsSvYMyGs63yzb1dTBF2JT~egsrL3zz
4Aoxf3NCAtwLTPSxRjByrjMwgO4rH2xeB31NvJtwnYIhxf0fgX7MhCDSYdk-
l3pznALzuIufPGQTuqxg__&Key-Pair-Id=APKAJLOHF5GGSLRBV4ZA

Naeem, M. Y., & Ugur, S. (2019). Nutritional content and health benefits of eggplant. *Turkish Journal of Agriculture-Food Science and Technology*, 7, 31-36. https://agrifoodscience.com/index.php/TURJAF/article/view/3146/1457

Okwu, D. E. (2008). Citrus fruits: A rich source of phytochemicals and their roles in human health. *Int. J. Chem. Sci*, 6(2), 451-471. http://library.cofer.edu.vn/TLTK/T%C3%A0i%20li%E1%BB%87u%20tham%20kh%E1%BA%A3o/BB_Citrus%20Fruits-%20A%20Rich%20Source%20of%20Phytochemicals%20and%20their%20Roles%20in%20Human%20Health_21tr%20(1)%20(1).pdf

Rahman, A. (2013). Health benefits, chemistry and mechanism of Carica papaya a crowning glory. *Advances in Natural Science*, 6(3), 26-37. https://d1wqtxts1xzle7.cloudfront.net/73421159/5167-libre.pdf?1634939202=&response-content-disposition=inline%3B+filename%3DHealth_Benefits_Chemistry_and_Mechanism.pdf&Expires=1704503218&Signature=WbacjFS0I33E99VyosAoGDJ8qNgZeuyYhYZn7AJk~A3rsA0eMvUhxm2Xf9~J2JMTIuA-xXdFjaB5dxDQUI5rSaa5bq5Oxu-3UhMbvBhvUnKq2q~jGxYtAsvEihG2nnHt6qfFHU~VRWt0TxbStKWiWvQDfC3eKMt~PlLIyRPNJfPVKW~lp8e-imzEGLgGLEz8JSt-eSkjL5eY-lUojKVQowgvtSYv0TqAKnXm~ajTvIJKFGp4nJuCRauwrUyI47v5Am249dY5trKyFJcNK0VqI4nS2a894EHW43FGyWmvS7Qz2lB4-~eoWF6hZgnKrzF89JdE-t9Xn0qRCPrItk6g9g__&Key-Pair-Id=APKAJLOHF5GGSLRBV4ZA

Rao, A. V., & Snyder, D. M. (2010). Raspberries and human health: a review. *Journal of Agricultural and Food Chemistry*, 58(7), 3871-3883. https://pubs.acs.org/doi/abs/10.1021/jf903484g

Reiland, H., & Slavin, J. (2015). Systematic review of pears and health. *Nutrition today*, 50(6), 301. https://www.ncbi.nlm.nih.gov/pmc/articles/PMC4657810/

Sharma, V., Sharma, L., & Sandhu, K. S. (2020). Cucumber (Cucumis sativus L.). *Antioxidants in vegetables and nuts-Properties and health benefits*, 333-340. https://www.researchgate.net/profile/Reshu-Rajput/publication/346530214_Pistachio/links/64d1efa691fb036ba6d623ad/Pistachio.pdf#page=338

Singh, B., Singh, J. P., Kaur, A., & Singh, N. (2016). Bioactive compounds in banana and their associated health benefits–A review. *Food chemistry*, *206*, 1-11. https://www.phytojournal.com/archives/2012/vol1issue3/PartA/9.1.pdf

Singh, J., Jayaprakasha, G. K., & Patil, B. S. (2018). Extraction, identification, and potential health benefits of spinach flavonoids: a review. *Advances in Plant Phenolics: From Chemistry to Human Health*, 107-136. https://drive.google.com/file/d/1HPptETAmIeFMxlcvPCP7BRcbV43JFboO/view

Tejada, L., Buendía-Moreno, L., Villegas, A., Cayuela, J. M., Bueno-Gavilá, E., Gómez, P., & Abellán, A. (2020). Nutritional and sensorial characteristics of zucchini (Cucurbita pepo L.) as affected by freezing and the culinary treatment. *International Journal of Food Properties*, *23*(1), 1825-1833.https://www.tandfonline.com/doi/pdf/10.1080/10942912.2020.1826512

Tsai, C. W., Chen, H. W., Sheen, L. Y., & Lii, C. K. (2012). Garlic: Health benefits and actions. *BioMedicine*, *2*(1), 17-29.https://d1wqtxts1xzle7.cloudfront.net/74826689/j.biomed.2011.12.00220211118-16718-ys6eao-libre.pdf?1637229723=&response-content-disposition=inline%3B+filename%3DGarlic_Health_benefits_and_actions.pdf&Expires=1705612152&Signature=BJt3Z3FUh9Vh6imcMf4kKPgh5rGf0Jcs1YTkPi1mfBps7JgJoM6vnZtg3foPbbj3LWfQ~V~CDptQU4JIKQkhsFfZS0zqXJyfb42-z8Tgtx4M1mdVBWU2kyzD~pHlVjKh-qkVFyHf7TN2dyYMWALreKq8YDp5EEHcqkfQGqykd-EIFQnO3YATNo2nhbWIz~5dUIcsrSHD4d4m5uHjTYipJ-QFIk4nRJad47E~26jzQk8V27XpmBduuEwHWY5cqFpbnRI9g8gsZo2uO8Iisynsva6YaC0ys~ETD46z3DfYAZ0CdByouBg323gLL7Wu8s1bYhPsj7XPTQElQEhDyme26Q__&Key-Pair-Id=APKAJLOHF5GGSLRBV4ZA

Tulipani, S., Mezzetti, B., & Battino, M. (2009). Impact of strawberries on human health: insight into marginally discussed bioactive compounds for the Mediterranean diet. *Public health nutrition*, *12*(9A), 1656-1662. https://www.cambridge.org/core/journals/public-health-nutrition/article/impact-of-strawberries-on-human-health-insight-into-marginally-discussed-bioactive-compounds-for-the-mediterranean-diet/7A7BCCCAEDE36ED4CB0185A19E2EC720

Tyagi, S., Nanher, A. H., Sahay, S., Kumar, V., Bhamini, K., Nishad, S. K., & Ahmad, M. (2015). Kiwifruit: Health benefits and medicinal importance. *Rashtriya krishi*, *10*(2), 98-100.

USDA. (2020) FoodData Central. https://fdc.nal.usda.gov/fdc-app.html#/

Varshney, K., & Mishra, K. (2022). An analysis of health benefits of carrot. International Journal of Innovative Research in Engineering & Management (IJIREM), 9, 211-214.https://www.researchgate.net/profile/Kirti-Mishra-9/publication/359863991_An_Analysis_of_Health_Benefits_of_Carrot/links/626914028e6d637bd1024749/An-Analysis-of-Health-Benefits-of-Carrot.pdf

Walia, A., Kumar, N., Singh, R., Kumar, H., Kumar, V., Kaushik, R., & Kumar, A. P. (2022). Bioactive compounds in Ficus fruits, their bioactivities, and associated health benefits: a review. *Journal of Food Quality*, *2022*, 1-19. https://www.hindawi.com/journals/jfq/2022/6597092/

Wu, Y., Han, T., Yang, H., Lyu, L., Li, W., & Wu, W. (2023). Known and potential health benefits and mechanisms of blueberry anthocyanins: A review. *Food Bioscience*, 103050.